# Enterovirus- D68:
## Tips to Keep Your
## Family Safe

# Enterovirus- D68:
# Tips to Keep Your
# Family Safe

by
## M. Taureen, PhD, MS

To all of the families whose lives are being devastated by the loss of a child and the spread of the 2014 Enterovirus D68.

_____

# Table of Contents

# Foreward

"Children are our most valuable resource."

~Herbert Hoover, 31st U.S. president

# Preface

This book was written to help parents and family members understand Enterovirus-68 and how to help keep the children in your family safe from this potentially deadly virus.

# Call to Action

Please follow these basic steps to keep your child from getting and spreading EV-D68!

# Introduction

Every year, millions of children in the United States catch enteroviruses that can cause coughing, sneezing, and fever. This year, the enterovirus that is most commonly causing respiratory illness in children across the country is enterovirus-D68 (EV-D68).

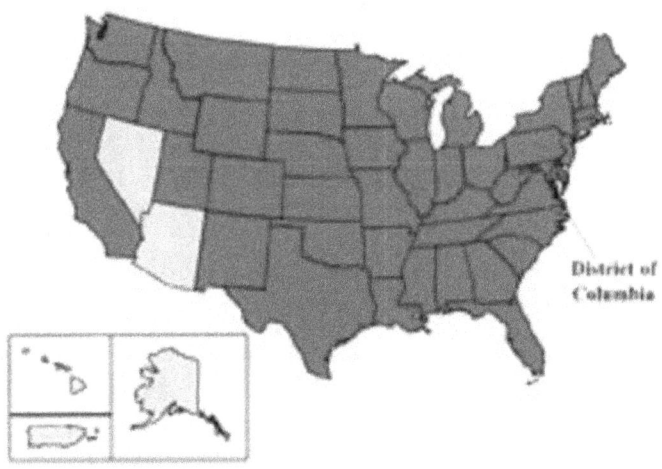

District of Columbia

*Image courtesy of http://www.cdc.gov/non-polio-enterovirus/EV-D68-outbreaks.html*

From mid-August to October 10, 2014, a total of 691 people in 46 states and the District of Columbia have been confirmed to have respiratory illness caused enterovirus-D68 (EV-D68).

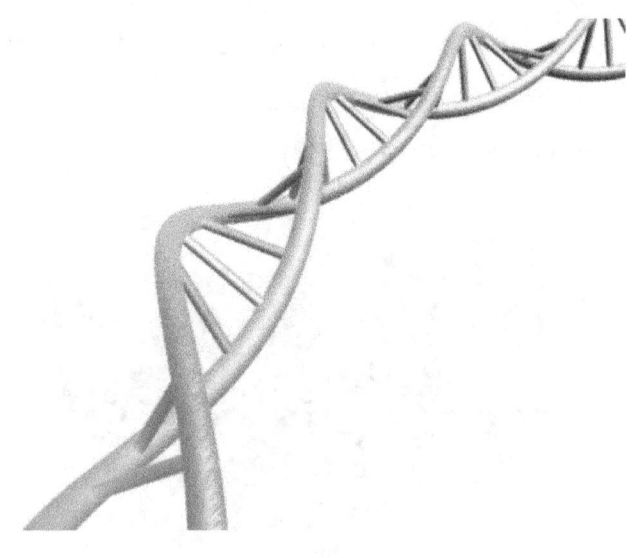

*IMAGE COURTESY OF COOLDESIGN AT FREEDIGITALPHOTOS.NET*

# Chapter 1

# What is an enterovirus?

Enteroviruses (EV) are common viruses and there are over 100 types. They are classified as RNA viruses which include those that polio and hepatitis A.

EV typically occurs in the gastrointestinal tract,  and can spread to the central nervous system or other parts of the body. EV generally affects millions of people worldwide each year, and are often found in the respiratory secretions (e.g., saliva, sputum, or nasal mucus) and stool of an infected person.

It is estimated that roughly  10-15 million EV infections occur in the U.S. per year. People are more likely to get infected with EV infections in the summer and fall.

This fact that the enteroviruses are of the RNA virus family means that they can mutate faster than other types of viruses. For this reason it's spread is not easily predicted and different strains of EV can be common in different years.

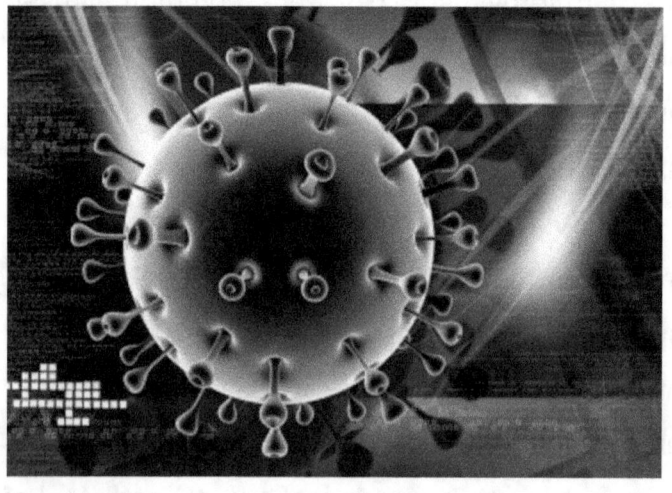

IMAGE COURTESY OF DREAM DESIGNS AT FREEDIGITALPHOTOS.NET

# Chapter 2

# What makes Enterovirus D68 (EV-D68) different?

Enterovirus D68 (EV-D68) is by no means a new virus, but historically it's far less common than other enteroviruses. EV-D68 was originally identified in California in 1962. Compared to other enteroviruses, EV-D68 has been least reported in the United States for the last 4 decades.

Recently, however there has been an increase in the EV-D68 strain. In 2014, there have been several childhood deaths directly linked to EV-D68.

EV-D68 is making people sick in almost all states. Most of the cases have been among children. EV-D68 can cause serious respiratory symptoms. It can be particularly serious for children with asthma or other respiratory conditions that make breathing difficult. For these children, EV-D68 infections can result in hospitalization and even death.

# Chapter 3

# How is Enterovirus D68 (EV-D68) Spread?

EV-D68 is spread through close contact with infected people. The virus likely spreads from person to person when an infected person coughs or sneezes. You can also become infected by touching objects or surfaces that have the virus on them and then touching your mouth, nose or eyes.

Enteroviruses are also present in stool and can be passed on to others when people do not wash their hands after touching stool.

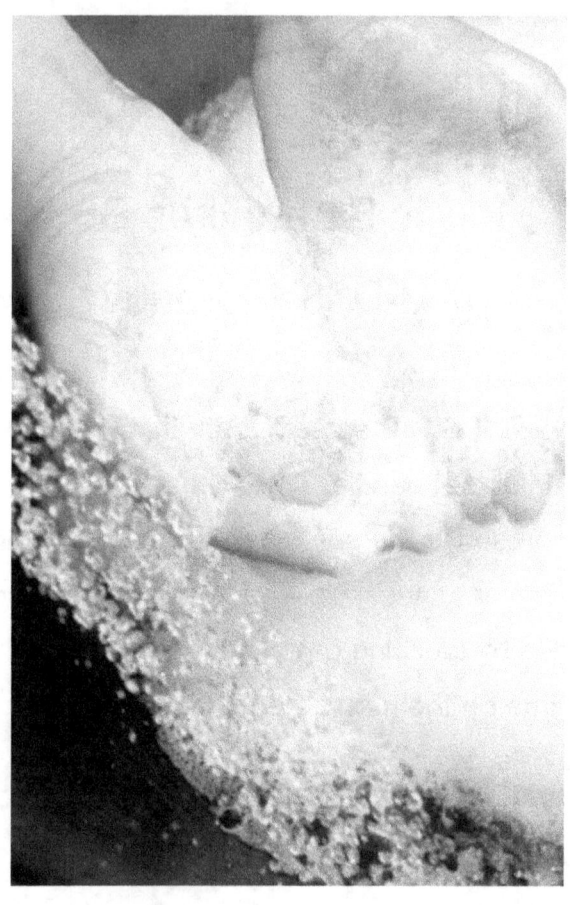

IMAGE COURTESY OF JACKTHUMM AT FREEDIGITALPHOTOS.NET

# Chapter 4

# Who is at Risk? What are the Risk Factors?

Infections with enteroviruses are usually common in the United States during summer and fall. Most people who get infected are infants, children and teens. In 2014 beginning in mid-August, states started seeing far more children in hospitals with severe respiratory illness caused by EV-D68. Since then, more testing has been done fore this particular strain. EV-D68 is making people sick in almost all states.

Anyone can get EV-D68, however, among the recent EV-D68 infections, children with asthma seemed to have a higher risk for severe respiratory symptoms.

Children are at higher risk for EV-D68. Infants, children, and teenagers are at higher risk than adults for getting infected and sick with enteroviruses like EV-D68. That's because they have not been exposed to these types of viruses before, and they do not yet have immunity (protection) built up to fight the disease. If your child has asthma, he or she may be at greater risk for severe respiratory illness from EV-D68.

Children less than 5 years old and children with pre-existing respiratory issues appear to be most at risk for the illness and severe symptoms. Also, illness in adults with asthma and those who are immunosuppressed have also been reported.

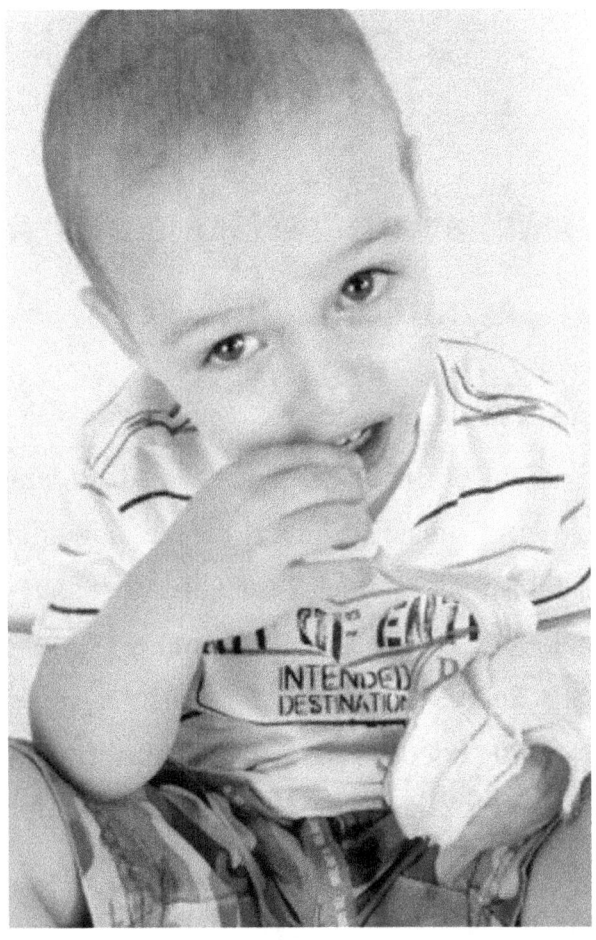

IMAGE COURTESY OF IMAGERYMAJESTIC AT
FREEDIGITALPHOTOS.NET

# Chapter 5

# What are the Signs and Symptoms of EV-68?

EV-D68 usually causes mild to severe respiratory illness; however, the full spectrum of EV-D68 illness is not well-defined. Most start with common cold symptoms of runny nose and cough. Some, but not all, may also have fever. For more severe cases, difficulty breathing, wheezing or problems catching your breath may occur.

**Mild symptoms** may include:
- Fever
- runny nose
- Sneezing
- Cough

- Body Aches
- Muscle aches

**Severe symptoms** may include:

- All symptoms included in mild presentation
- wheezing
- difficulty breathing.

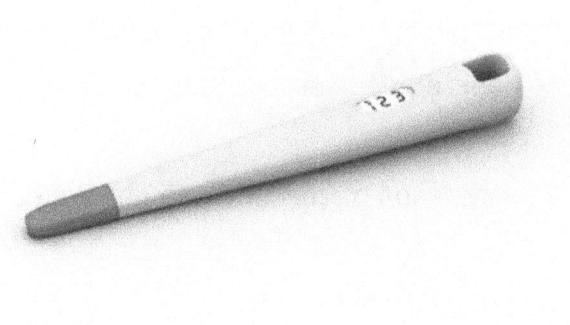

IMAGE COURTESY OF RENJITH KRISHNAN AT
FREEDIGITALPHOTOS.NET

# Chapter 6

# How do you protect your family from EV-D68?

To help avoid catching and spreading EV-D68, parents and children should always follow these basic steps to stay healthy :

- Wash hands often with soap and water for 20 seconds.
- Washing hands correctly is the most important thing you can do to stay healthy.
- Avoid touching eyes, nose and mouth with unwashed hands.
- Avoid close contact, such as kissing, hugging, and sharing cups or eating utensils, with people who are sick.

- Cover your coughs and sneezes with a tissue or shirt sleeve, not your hands.
- Clean and disinfect frequently touched surfaces, such as toys and doorknobs, especially if someone is sick.

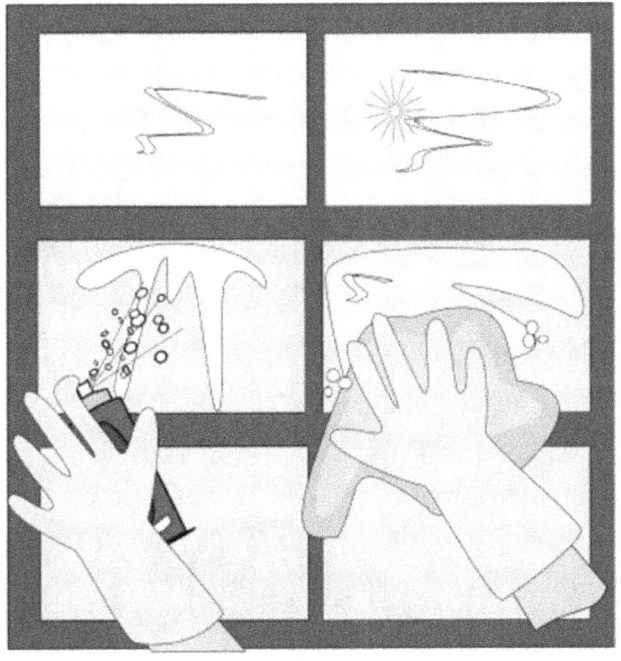

IMAGE COURTESY OF DEBSPOONS AT FREEDIGITALPHOTOS.NET

# Chapter 7

# Does your child or teenager have asthma or any other respiratory condition?

Its better to be safe rather than sorry! Children with asthma are particularly at risk for severe symptoms from EV-D68 infection.

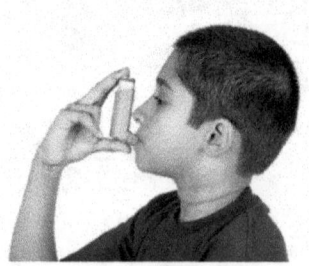

IMAGE COURTESY OF ARVIND BALARAMAN AT
FREEDIGITALPHOTOS.NET

Therefore, if your child has asthma, take some precautionary measures to be prepared in the event that he or she catches EV-D68. Recommendations are to:

- Discuss and update your child's asthma action plan with his or her doctor.
- Make sure your child takes his or her prescribed asthma medications as directed, especially long-term control medication(s).
- Make sure your child knows to keep asthma reliever medication with him or her or has access to it at all times.
- Get your child a flu vaccine, since flu and other respiratory infections can trigger an asthma attack.
- If your child develops new or worsening asthma symptoms, follow the steps of his or her asthma action plan.
- If symptoms do not go away, call your child's doctor right away.

- Make sure caregiver(s) and/or teacher(s) are aware of the child's condition, and that they know how to help if the child experiences any symptoms related to asthma.
- Call your child's doctor if he or she is having difficulty breathing, if you feel you are unable to control symptoms, or if symptoms are getting worse.

# Chapter 8

# Do you suspect that a child has contracted EV-D68?

If your child is displaying symptoms of EV-68 call your medical provider as soon as possible! Please keep your child out of school or daycare for the safety of other children. As expressed before it is better to be safe rather than sorry.

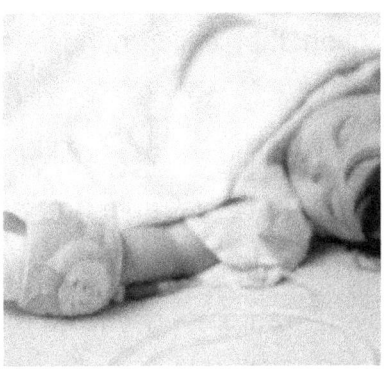

IMAGE COURTESY OF JOMPHONG AT FREEDIGITALPHOTOS.NET

# Chapter 9

# Is there is a treatment, cure or vaccine for EV-68?

NO! There is no specific treatment for EV-D68. There is no vaccine for EV-D68 infection. The best cure at this point is prevention. This particular strain of virus has become easier to spread this year and also there may not be as much protection that children have against this particular strain

If your child has mild respiratory symptoms, you may be able to relieve some symptoms with over-the-counter medicine for pain and fever. Remember, children **should not** be given aspirin. Talk to your child's doctor about the best way to control his or her symptoms.

# Chapter 10

# Has your child been diagnosed with EV or EV-D68?

If a child is diagnosed with EV or EV-D68 its is best to keep them school or daycare. Children without a fever should be monitored until symptom free. Children with a fever (oral temperature of >100°F) must stay home until they are fever-free for 24 hours without fever-reducing medication.

As with other respiratory infections, including the flu and the common cold, there is some increase in risk of catching EV-D68 in places with large numbers of people, such as schools and daycare settings.

Children can protect themselves and others by:

- washing their hands often
- not touching their eyes and noses
- coughing or sneezing into a tissue or their arm/elbow
- properly disposing of the tissue

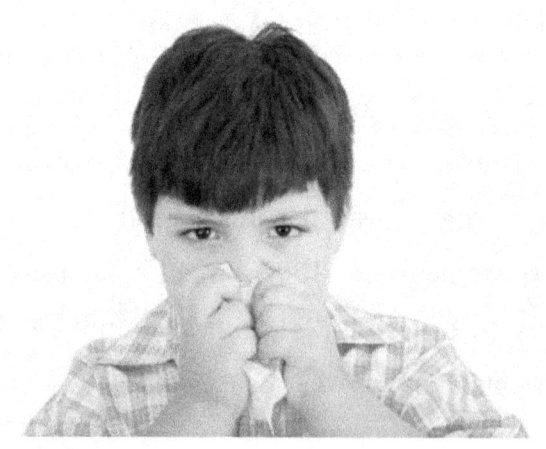

IMAGE COURTESY OF DAVID CASTILLO DOMINICI AT
FREEDIGITALPHOTOS.NET

# Chapter 11

# Do you want more information about EV-D68?

➤ For more information about EV-D68 speak with your medical provider

➤ You can also find helpful links at:

  ➤ *The Centers for Disease Control and Prevention:* http://www.cdc.gov

  ➤ *Your Local Public Health Department*